PARKISON'S, NOW WHAT?

By Daniel Funderburg

"Parkinson's, Now What? *A Guide for the Newly Diagnosed*"

Chapter 1: Understanding Parkinson's: An Overview

- Clear and simple explanation of what Parkinson's disease is.
- Overview of common symptoms and how they may manifest.

Chapter 2: Your Care Team

- Introduction to the healthcare professionals and support members who will be part of the Parkinson's care team.

Chapter 3: Living Well with Parkinson's: Lifestyle Adjustments

- Practical tips for maintaining a healthy lifestyle despite the diagnosis.
- Introduction to the role of exercise, nutrition, and sleep in managing Parkinson's.

Chapter 4: Medications and Treatment Options

- Overview of common medications prescribed for Parkinson's.
- Explanation of treatment options and potential side effects.

Chapter 5: Daily Living Strategies

- Practical advice for adapting daily routines to make life with Parkinson's more manageable.
- Tips for maintaining independence and quality of life.

Chapter 6: Emotional Well-being

- Addressing the emotional impact of a Parkinson's diagnosis.
- Encouragement to seek support and engage in activities that promote mental health.

Chapter 7: Building a Support System

- The importance of family, friends, and community in coping with Parkinson's.
- Tips for communicating with loved ones about the diagnosis.

Chapter 8: Resources and Advocacy

- Introduction to resources available for individuals with Parkinson's.
- Advocacy tips and guidance for accessing support networks.

Chapter 9: Looking Ahead: Hope and Positivity

- Encouragement to maintain a positive outlook on life with Parkinson's.
- Stories of individuals who have successfully navigated life after a Parkinson's diagnosis.

I know that finding out you have Parkinson's disease can be a difficult and upsetting experience. It is important to first accept the wide range of feelings you may be experiencing now, including anxiety, uncertainty, and even a sense of loss. It is acceptable to allow yourself the time and space to process these emotions in your own way because these feelings are perfectly normal.

Parkinson's disease presents a distinct set of difficulties, but it is crucial that you understand this illness does not define you. You remain the same person with aspirations, passions, and an abundance of life experiences that shape who you are. There is much more to your story than Parkinson's disease; it is only one part of your story.

Remember, there are many resources at your fingertips to help you through this new phase. The best support and attention will be given to you by a group called your care team. Together, you will create a plan that specifically takes care of your needs and concerns.

The Parkinson's community also has many people who are willing to share their stories, encourage one another, and offer insightful advice. Making connections with people who have experienced circumstances like this can be comforting and empowering. To share your journey and get insight from others' experiences, think about contacting nearby support groups or online forums.

Always remember that it is ok to rely on your loved ones for support and comfort. Friends and family can be invaluable partners on this journey, providing the emotional support needed during transition times and offering helpful advice.

You can find a wide range of resources to assist you in adjusting to life with Parkinson's disease, including educational materials and symptom management tips. Remember knowledge gives you power and starts every day out toward building a life that is fulfilling and rewarding.

Above all, remember to treat yourself with kindness. You are not expected to know everything at once; this is a journey. Allow yourself to grow, change, and find new aspects of your journey to look forward to too.

As you embark on this journey, please remember that hope is a powerful force. There are ongoing advancements in research and treatments for Parkinson's, and the future holds the promise of progress and improved quality of life.

You have the strength and ability to handle this problem with dignity and grace because you are resilient. Take it one step at a time and remember that you are surrounded by caring people!

Ok so we have received the diagnoses of Parkinson's, now what? Let us break down Parkinson's disease and its impact on daily life in easy-to-understand terms so we do not get overwhelmed!

Understanding Parkinson's Disease:

Parkinson's disease is a condition that affects the brain. In simple terms, it happens when certain cells in your brain stop working correctly. These cells are responsible for producing a chemical called dopamine, which helps control movements and coordination throughout your body.

Impact on Daily Life:

1. **Movement Challenges:**
   - People with Parkinson's may experience tremors or shaking in their hands, making it harder to perform tasks like holding a cup, cell phone or writing.

- Stiffness in muscles can make movements slow and rigid, affecting activities like walking or getting up from a chair. Doctors will call this Rigidity!

2. **Balance and Coordination:**

    - Parkinson's can affect balance, making it more challenging to stay steady on your feet. This might increase the risk of falls.

3. **Fine Motor Skills:**

    - Tasks that require precise hand movements, like buttoning a shirt or tying shoelaces, can become more difficult.

4. **Facial Expressions:**

    - Some individuals with Parkinson's may have a reduced range of facial expressions, which can impact communication.

5. **Speech Changes:**
   - Parkinson's can affect the muscles used for speaking, leading to softer or more monotone speech.

6. **Fatigue:**
   - People with Parkinson's may feel more tired than usual, even after doing simple activities.

7. **Emotional Impact:**
   - Dealing with changes in daily life can be emotionally challenging. It is common to feel frustrated, anxious, or even depressed.

Managing Strategies:

1. **Medications:**
   - There are medications that can help manage symptoms and improve quality of life.

2. **Exercise:**
   - Physical activity, especially exercises that improve balance and flexibility, can be beneficial.

3. **Adapting your Environment:**
   - Making changes at home, like adding handrails or using adaptive tools, like reaching aids, can make daily tasks easier.

4. **Speech and Physical Therapy:**
   - These therapies can provide techniques to enhance communication and movement.

5. **Support System:**
    - Having a dedicated support system, including family, friends, and healthcare professionals, is crucial.

It is critical to keep in mind that, despite the difficulties caused by Parkinson's disease, lifestyle adjustment and management solutions exist. Maintaining a fulfilling life can be easier by asking for help when needed and continuing participating in enjoyable activities. Always seek the advice of healthcare professionals for specific therapy and guidance.

Understanding Parkinson's: An Overview

Parkinson's disease is a neurological (brain) condition that primarily affects movement and memory. Named after James Parkinson, the British physician who first described the symptoms in 1817, this chronic disorder gradually progresses over time. While there is currently no cure for Parkinson's, there are various treatments available to manage its symptoms and improve the quality of life for those affected.

What is Parkinson's Disease?

At its core, Parkinson's is characterized by the malfunction and gradual loss of nerve cells, or neurons, in a part of the brain called the substantia nigra. These neurons are responsible for producing dopamine, a neurotransmitter that plays a crucial role in transmitting signals within the brain to control movement and coordination.

The reduction in dopamine levels results in the hallmark symptoms of Parkinson's, which primarily affect movement. While the exact cause of Parkinson's remains unknown, genetic, and environmental factors are believed to contribute to its development.

Common Symptoms and Manifestations:

1. **Tremors (shaky hands)**:

    One of the most noticeable signs is trembling, or uncontrollably shaking, which usually starts in the hands or fingers. These tremors might happen when you are moving and when you are at rest.

2. **Bradykinesia (slow motion movements):**

    The word "bradykinesia" describes slow movement. Parkinson's patients may find it difficult to start and finish everyday tasks, which can cause a noticeable slowing in their overall movement.

3. **Muscle Rigidity (stiff muscles):**

One common sign is stiffness or rigidity in the muscles, which makes it difficult for people to bend and stretch their arms and legs smoothly.

4. **Postural Instability (balance):**

This may affect coordination and balance, which increases the possibility of falls. Individuals could experience uneasiness or struggle to keep their posture straight.

5. **Tiny Handwriting (micrographia):**

Individuals with Parkinson's may notice a decrease in the size of their handwriting, and the writing itself may appear cramped.

6. **Masked Face (facial movements):**

    People with Parkinson's disease may appear to be less animated due to reduced facial expressions, also known as a "masked face," even when they are feeling a wide range of emotions.

7. **Speech Changes (sounds different):**

    - Changes in speech patterns, such as softer or monotone speech, may occur. Individuals may find it challenging to say words clearly.

8. **Freezing Episodes (frozen movements):**

    - Some people with Parkinson's may experience "freezing," where they temporarily feel as though their feet are glued to the ground, making it difficult to initiate movement.

It is important to remember that each person will experience signs differently, as will how they develop. Parkinson's disease can impact non-motor functions as well, which can result in problems including mood disorders, difficulty sleeping, and dementia, among other things, even though movement-related symptoms are the most well-known.

Knowledge empowers people with Parkinson's disease as well as those who support them. Parkinson's patients continue to have hope for better medicines and a better future because of advancements in research and treatment.

Chapter 2: Your Parkinson's Team

Welcome to your Parkinson's team! These are the special people who will help you on your journey. Let us meet them and learn why talking with them is super important.

1. Neurologist - The Brain Boss:

Imagine your brain is like a city, and the neurologist is the mayor. They understand how Parkinson's affects the brain and make plans to help you feel better.

2. Movement Specialist - The Motion Expert:

The movement specialist is like a coach for your body. They know tricks to make your movements smoother.

3. Physical Therapist - The Exercise Guru:

Meet your exercise guru, the physical therapist. They have fun exercises to keep your body strong and flexible, like a workout coach just for you.

4. Speech Therapist - The Word Wizard:

The word wizard, or speech therapist, helps you talk clearly and loudly. They have cool exercises and tips to keep your voice strong.

5. Occupational Therapist - The Daily Life Helper:

An occupational therapist is like a helper for your everyday tasks. They find cool ways to make things easier, from making a cup of coffee, to getting a shower to getting dressed for the day.

6. Your Personal Support Person(s):

The friends or family who step up and walk with you step by step on your new journey. Always around to help you understand, work on, and talk about your journey.

Why Do You Need All These People?

Now, let us talk about why telling your healthcare team everything is important.

1. Share Your Feelings:

If you are feeling happy, sad, or anything in between, tell your care team. They are here for you, your body, and your feelings.

2. Talk About Changes:

If something feels different or new, let them know. They can change the plan to help you better, like adjusting a strategy during a game.

3. Ask Questions:

Ask questions about your treatment, medicine, or anything on your mind. The more you understand, the more powerful you become in your journey.

4. Bring Your Sidekicks (Family and Friends):

Your family and friends are also part of your care team. Bring them to appointments and share what you notice. More eyes and ears mean more support and help.

Remember, your team is here to make you the hero of your story. By talking openly, you make a super team that beats Parkinson's together.

Chapter 3: Living Well with Parkinson's: Lifestyle Adjustments

In this chapter, we will learn practical tips for maintaining a healthy lifestyle despite the diagnosis and discover the roles of exercise, nutrition, and sleep in managing Parkinson's.

1. Practical Tips

Create a Daily Routine:

- Imagine your day planned out before the day. Having a
- consistent schedule can make things more predictable and manageable, which helps create less stress.

Stay Socially Active:

- Joining clubs or spending time with friends is beneficial for your physical and mental health. Socializing can lift your spirits and create a great support network.

Mindful Relaxation:

- Picture a calm lake in your mind. Practices like meditation or deep breathing can be your magical spell to relax and reduce stress.

2. The Medicine of Exercise:

Workout:

- Think of exercise as you would taking a daily medicine. It keeps your body strong. Activities like walking, yoga, elastic band training, even doing household chores can create increased strength, balance, and flexibility.

Balance Training:

- Balance exercises are training your body to prevent falls and keeping you steady.

3. Nutrition: Fueling your Life:

Healthy Ingredients:

- Eating a balanced diet is like using magical ingredients. Include fruits, vegetables, whole grains, and proteins to keep your body fueled.

Hydration:

- Water is your magic potion for staying hydrated. It helps your body and mind function at its best.

4. **The Rejuvenation of Good Sleep:**

Sleep Well:

- Quality sleep is your goal for rejuvenation. Ensure a comfortable sleep environment and maintain a consistent sleep schedule.

Limiting Caffeine and Screens:

- Imagine turning off all gadgets and television before bedtime. Limiting caffeine and screen time helps you relax and fall into a deep, restful sleep.

5. **Be Mindful:**

   Mental Exercises:

   - Imagine your brain as a library. Engage in activities like puzzles, games, or reading to keep your mind sharp.

   Positivity:

   - Surround yourself with positivity. Whether it is through hobbies, music, or spending time with loved ones, these are your magical charms against negativity.

Embracing and incorporating these lifestyle practices, you will discover the secret to living well with Parkinson's – a life filled with fulfillment, strength, and joy.

Chapter 4: Medication and Treatment: Choosing the Right Path

In this chapter, we will delve into the world of medications and treatment options for Parkinson's. Do not let it overwhelm you! Let us explore together the common medications, understand the different treatment approaches, and be aware of potential side effects.

1. Common Medications:

Levodopa: (Energy Booster):

- Levodopa is a key medication that boosts energy levels by converting into dopamine, helping improve movement.

Dopamine Agonists: (Mimics Dopamine):

- Dopamine agonists mimic the effects of dopamine, assisting in managing movement symptoms.

- **MAO-B Inhibitors: (Protects Dopamine):**
  - These inhibitors protect dopamine, ensuring its prolonged effectiveness in managing symptoms.

COMT Inhibitors: (Enhances Levodopa):
  - COMT inhibitors enhance the effects of levodopa, extending its benefits.

2. Treatment Options:

Deep Brain Stimulation (DBS): (Internal Help):
  - DBS involves sending signals to the brain internally, reducing symptoms and restoring balance.

Physical and Occupational Therapy: (Getting Stronger)

- Therapy helps maintain physical strength and enhances overall mobility.

Speech Therapy: (Clear Communication):

- Speech therapy focuses on maintaining clear communication, addressing any challenges in your speech.

3. Potential Side Effects:

Nausea and Dizziness: (Something is not right):

- Some medications may cause nausea or dizziness. It is important to discuss any discomfort with your care team.

Sleep Disturbances: (Change in sleep):

- Certain medications might impact sleep patterns. If you

experience changes, inform your care team for guidance.

Impulsive Behavior: (Noticing Changes):

- Rarely, medications may lead to impulsive behavior. It is crucial to monitor any unusual changes and communicate them to your care team.

4. Crafting Your Treatment Plan:

Consulting Your Healthcare Provider and Care Team: Creating a Plan:

- Regular consultations with your healthcare provider and care team are essential for creating and adjusting your treatment plan.

Open Communication: Sharing Experiences:

- Openly sharing your experiences and any

concerns with your healthcare provider and care team ensures a collaborative approach to managing your Parkinson's.

Understanding the array of medications, treatment options, and potential side effects empowers you to actively participate in your Parkinson's journey. With a well-crafted treatment plan and effective communication, you can navigate the path towards optimal wellness.

Chapter 5: Daily Living Tips: Life with Parkinson's

In this chapter, we will explore practical advice and tips to for daily routines, making life with Parkinson's more manageable. Discover tips for maintaining independence and enhancing your overall quality of life.

1. Daily Routines:

Establish a Consistent Routine:

- Creating a consistent daily routine provides a sense of predictability and makes tasks more manageable.

Prioritize Tasks:

- Prioritizing tasks helps focus on what needs to be done first, preventing you becoming overwhelmed and stressed.

Break Tasks into Smaller Steps:

- Breaking down activities into smaller steps makes them more achievable and less daunting.

2. Mobility and Independence:

Living Spaces:

- Adapt your living spaces for accessibility, considering features like handrails, walkers, wheelchairs, and proper lighting.

Mobility Aids:

- Explore the use of mobility aids such as canes or walkers to enhance stability and independence.

Assist Devices:

- Devices for daily tasks, such as jar openers or specialized utensils, to make everyday activities more manageable.

3. Communication Strategies:

Speak Clearly and Slowly:

- Speaking clearly and at a slower pace improves communication, ensuring your message is effectively conveyed.

Use Visual Aids:

- Visual aids, like calendars, dry erase boards and reminder boards, assist in organizing daily schedules and activities.

Expressing Needs:

- Clearly expressing your needs and preferences helps others understand how to provide the support you need and want.

4. Embracing Technological Assistance:

Smart Devices and Apps:

- Explore the use of smart devices and applications to set reminders, manage schedules, and stay organized.

Voice-Activated Technology:

- Voice-activated technology can simplify tasks, allowing for hands-free control of various devices.

5. Emotions:

Engage in Hobbies and Interests:

- Pursuing hobbies and interests contributes to emotional well-being, providing joy and fulfillment.

Connect with Supportive Networks:

- Established connections with support groups and networks are in your community to share experiences and gain valuable insights.

Seek Professional Support:

- Professional support, such as counseling or therapy, can provide support for emotional challenges.

6. Quality of Life Tips:

Prioritize Self-Care (you come first):

- Prioritizing self-care activities, whether it is reading, enjoying nature, or coloring daily activities will help you stay emotionally positive.

Celebrate Achievements:

- Celebrate small achievements to acknowledge progress and maintain a positive outlook.

By incorporating these daily living strategies, you empower yourself to navigate the challenges of Parkinson's while preserving your independence and enriching your quality of life. Each change contributes to a more manageable and fulfilling daily experience.

Chapter 6: Emotional Well-being: Nurturing You

In this chapter, we will talk about emotional well-being and explore ways to address the impact of a Parkinson's diagnosis. We will look for encouragement to seek support and engage in activities that promote mental health, remember it is all about you!

1. Acknowledging the Diagnosis:

Your Feelings:

- Acknowledge the range of emotions that may accompany a Parkinson's diagnosis, from uncertainty to resilience to anger and being scared, they are all normal feelings.

Your Response:

- Recognize that experiencing a mix of emotions is a normal part of the journey, and it is okay to feel a variety of emotions that change, even minute by minute.

2. Building a Support System:

Connecting with Loved Ones:

- Strengthen connections with family and friends, sharing your feelings and allowing them to provide support.

Joining Support Groups:

- Explore support groups within the Parkinson's community to connect with individuals facing similar challenges, fostering a sense of understanding and teamwork.

Professional Guidance:

- Seek the guidance of mental health professionals, such as counselors or therapists, for personalized support and coping strategies.

3. Engaging in Mental Health Activities:

Mindfulness and Meditation:

- Start meditation practices to cultivate a sense of peace and reduce stress.

Artistic Expressions:

- Engage in artistic expressions, whether through painting, writing, coloring, or music, as a therapeutic outlet for your emotions and strengthening your mind.

Physical Exercise:

- Participate in regular physical exercise, known for its positive impact on mood and overall mental well-being. Small exercises of any kind can be beneficial.

4. Resilience and Positivity:

Setting Realistic Goals:

- Establish realistic goals and celebrate even small achievements, fostering a sense of accomplishment.

Positivity:

- Embrace a positive mindset by focusing on what you can control, gratitude, and finding joy in daily life and activities.

Adapting to Change:

- Develop resilience by adapting to the changes Parkinson's may bring, viewing challenges as opportunities for growth.

5. Prioritizing Self-Care:

Rest and Relaxation:

- Prioritize rest and relaxation, allowing time for rejuvenation and self-care.

Seeking Moments of Joy:

- Incorporate activities that bring moments of joy and fulfillment into your daily routine.

By tending to your emotional well-being like a garden, you can navigate the emotional landscape of Parkinson's with grace. Embrace the support around you, engage in activities that bring peace, and cultivate a positive mindset to nurture your emotions and thoughts and promote your overall emotional well-being.

Chapter 7: Building a Support System:

Strength in Connections

In this chapter, we will explore the significance of family, friends, and community in supporting you with Parkinson's. Discover valuable tips for communicating with loved ones about the diagnosis and building a robust support system for your journey.

1. The Power of Connections:

Family as Pillars of Support:

- Recognize the crucial role family plays as pillars of support. Share your experiences, fears, and triumphs with those closest to you.

Friends:

- Friends are like allies on your journey. Their understanding and encouragement contribute to a resilient support system.

Community:

- Connect with the broader Parkinson's community. Shared experiences and create bonds that inspire and uplift you and others.

2. Tips for Communicating the Diagnosis:

Choose the Right Time:

- Select a calm and private moment to share your diagnosis, allowing for an open and focused conversation.

Use Clear and Simple Language:

- Communicate using clear and simple language. Help your loved ones understand

Parkinson's without overwhelming them.

Express Your Emotions:

- Share your emotions openly. This creates an atmosphere of honesty and invites support.

3. Nurturing Open Communication:

Encourage Questions:

- Invite questions from your loved ones. It fosters open dialogue.

Express Your Needs:

- Clearly communicate your needs and preferences. This ensures your support system understands how to assist you effectively.

Share Treatment Plans:

- Keep your loved ones informed about your treatment plans. It helps them understand the journey ahead and how they can contribute.

4. Embracing Emotional Support:

Listening:

- Practice active listening and empathize with the emotions of your loved ones. Understanding is the foundation of strong emotional support.

Encouraging:

- Encourage your loved ones to express their feelings and concerns. This exchange will strengthen the bond of support.

Celebrating Achievements Together:

- Celebrate not only your achievements but the collective triumphs of your support system. It reinforces a positive and united approach.

5. Strengthening Bonds:

Regular Updates:

- Provide regular updates on your Parkinson's journey. This ongoing communication ensures your support system remains engaged and informed.

Inclusion in Decision-Making:

- Include your loved ones in decisions related to your health and well-being. Their involvement fosters a sense of shared responsibility.

Expressing Gratitude:

- Express gratitude for the unwavering support you receive. Acknowledging the efforts of your support system reinforces the strength of your connections.

Building a support system is like constructing a sturdy bridge for your Parkinson's journey. By fostering open communication, sharing your needs, and celebrating each step together, you create a network of strength that uplifts and empowers everyone involved.

Chapter 8: Resources: Empowering Your Journey

In this chapter, we will explore the vast array of resources available for individuals with Parkinson's. Additionally, we will investigate tips and guidance to help you access support networks and empower your journey.

1. Navigating Resources:

Educational:

- Discover a wealth of educational materials about Parkinson's. Books, websites, and informational pamphlets can offer valuable insights.

Support Organizations:

- Connect with Parkinson's support organizations. These groups provide a network of assistance, information, and understanding.

Local Support Groups:

- Explore local support groups in your community. Sharing experiences with others facing similar challenges can be incredibly uplifting.

2. Healthcare Team Collaboration:

Open Communication with Healthcare Team:

- Maintain open communication with your healthcare team. They are a crucial resource, guiding you through treatment options and providing personalized support.

Specialized Services:

- Investigate specialized services within your healthcare network, such as movement disorder clinics or therapists with expertise in Parkinson's care.

3. Financial Assistance and Planning:

Insurance Coverage:

- Familiarize yourself with your insurance coverage. Understanding the financial aspects of care is essential for planning and accessing necessary services.

Exploring Financial Aid Programs:

- Research financial aid programs and assistance available for individuals with Parkinson's. These programs can provide relief for medical expenses and related costs.

4. Legal and Employment Resources:

Legal Support Services:

- Consider seeking legal support services to navigate legal aspects related to

Parkinson's, such as creating advance directives.

Employment Resources:

- Explore resources related to employment and Parkinson's. Understanding workplace rights and available accommodations is crucial for maintaining employment.

5. Advocacy Tips:

Know Your Rights:

- Educate yourself about the rights of individuals with Parkinson's. Being informed empowers you to advocate effectively.

Communication:

- Practice effective communication when advocating for your needs. Clearly express your requirements and collaborate with your support team to achieve common goals.

Join Advocacy Groups:

- Participate in Parkinson's advocacy groups. These groups work collectively to raise awareness, influence policy changes, and enhance resources for the Parkinson's community.

6. Connecting:

National Parkinson's Foundations:

- Connect with national Parkinson's foundations. These organizations often lead advocacy efforts, providing a platform for your voice to be heard.

Community Engagement:

- Engage with local groups. Your involvement contributes

to the collective effort to improve resources and support for individuals with Parkinson's in your community.

Empowering your journey involves tapping into a rich tapestry of resources and advocating for the support you need. By navigating these avenues, you not only enhance your own experience but contribute to the broader efforts to improve the lives of those living with Parkinson's.

Chapter 9: Looking Ahead: Hope and Positivity

In this chapter, we get ready to embark on a journey filled with hope and positivity, exploring the encouragement to maintain a positive outlook on life with Parkinson's.

1. Positive Mindset:

The Power of Positivity:

- Explore the transformative power of a positive mindset. Embracing optimism can reshape your perspective and influence your journey with Parkinson's.

Resilience:

- Cultivate resilience as a tool to navigate challenges. Recognize the strength within you to overcome obstacles and emerge stronger.

2. Personal Narratives:

Voices of Resilience:

- Hear stories of resilience from individuals who have faced Parkinson's with courage. Their experiences offer inspiration and insights into navigating the path ahead.

Triumphs Over Challenges:

- Explore triumphs over challenges. Witness how individuals have found joy, purpose, and fulfillment despite the hurdles presented by Parkinson's.

Incorporating Joyful Activities:

- Learn how incorporating joyful activities into daily life contributes to a sense of happiness and satisfaction, fostering a positive environment.

4. Building a Supportive Community:

Community Bonds:

- Witness the strength of community bonds. Joining support groups and connecting with others creates a network of understanding and encouragement.

Shared Wisdom:

- Benefit from shared wisdom within the Parkinson's community. Discover insights and tips from those who have successfully navigated their journey.

5. Future Possibilities:

Parkinson's Research:

- Stay informed about advancements in Parkinson's research. Exciting possibilities and breakthroughs offer hope for improved treatments and a cure.

Living a Fulfilling Life:

- Explore the potential for living a fulfilling life with Parkinson's. As individuals share their stories, they envision a future filled with meaningful experiences and accomplishments.

6. Celebrating:

Marking Progress:

- Celebrate personal milestones and achievements. Recognizing progress, no matter how small, contributes to a positive narrative of growth and accomplishment.

Creating New Dreams:

- Encourage the creation of new dreams and aspirations. Life after a Parkinson's diagnosis is a canvas waiting for colorful expressions of hope and possibilities.

It is okay to have a range of emotions and expressing them is a brave step. Allow yourself the space to process and reach out whenever you need a listening ear or a comforting presence. There is strength in vulnerability, and your journey is a testament to resilience.

Remember, this diagnosis is just a chapter in your life, not the entire story. You have the power to shape your narrative, and there are countless possibilities waiting to unfold. Cherish the moments of joy, celebrate your achievements, and know that hope is a constant companion on this journey.

Parkinson's does not define you; it is just a part of your story. Embrace each day with the strength that resides within you and know that there is a community ready to stand by your side. Your courage in facing this challenge is remarkable, and I believe that, all of us together, we can navigate the road ahead.

As we venture into the future, let this small book serve as a beacon of hope and positivity. Through shared experiences, uplifting narratives, and a collective spirit, we embrace the limitless potential for a fulfilling and meaningful life with Parkinson's. The journey ahead is illuminated with hope, and the possibilities are as boundless as the human spirit.

www.ingramcontent.com/pod-product-compliance
Lightning Source LLC
Chambersburg PA
CBHW050243230526
45470CB00005B/2088